MORNING BANANA DIET GUIDE BOOK

Achieve Peak Health with the Morning Banana Diet: The Key to a Balanced Diet

REX LEWIS

Table of Contents

Introduction..................**5**

CHAPTER ONE **10**

The Inception of the Morning Banana Diet **10**

Preparing Mentally and Physically **13**

CHAPTER TWO **21**

Getting Started Morning Banana Diet **21**

The Banana as a Super food...**26**

CHAPTER THREE **32**

Nutritional Benefits **32**

Meal Planning **37**

CHAPTER FOUR..................**43**

Exercise and Physical Activity **43**

Overcoming Challenges..........**50**

Maintaining the Morning Banana Diet 58

Conclusion 65

THE END 68

Introduction

The Morning Banana Diet became a popular weight loss trend in Japan and subsequently gained favor in other regions. The diet was derived from the experiences of a Japanese couple, Sumiko Watanabe and her spouse Hitoshi Watanabe. The pair recorded their progress in losing weight, and the dietary regimen attracted significant public interest following its appearance on a popular Japanese social media platform.

The Morning Banana Diet is known for its straightforwardness and adaptability.

The diet is characterized by the following major features:

1. The primary element of the diet involves consuming one or more bananas as the morning meal. It is advisable to consume the bananas at ambient temperature and refrain from consuming any other food for breakfast. If you are still experiencing hunger, you may choose to delay your next meal for a period of 15 minutes, after which you are free to consume any food of your preference for the remaining meals.

2. Lunch and dinner: There are no rigid guidelines for lunch and dinner. Participants are recommended to consume a well-balanced and reasonable meal. The focus is on ceasing consumption when one experiences a sense of satisfaction rather than excessive fullness. The diet does not impose limitations on any particular food groups, rather it promotes conscientious and controlled consumption of food portions.

3. Avoid Consuming Snacks After 8 PM: The plan recommends refraining from eating snacks or meals late at night, and the final meal or snack should be had prior to 8 PM. This approach is said to provide the digestive system with sufficient time to relax during the night.

4. Hydration: It is advised to consume water regularly throughout the day, with a preference for water at room temperature or slightly warm.

5. Additional Recommendations: The diet also highlights the significance of obtaining an adequate amount of sleep, often targeting approximately 7-8 hours per night. In addition, it recommends abstaining from dairy and alcohol, and participating in low-intensity physical activity if preferred.

Although the Morning Banana Diet became famous due to its simplicity and the anecdotal success stories of its creators, it is important to acknowledge that outcomes may differ for each individual. Prior to making substantial alterations to your dietary habits, particularly if you have pre-existing health concerns, it is imperative to get guidance from a healthcare practitioner. It is advisable to prioritize total health and well-being when considering the Morning Banana Diet, rather than solely focusing on weight loss.

CHAPTER ONE
The Inception of the Morning Banana Diet

The Morning Banana Diet was first introduced in Japan and acquired extensive recognition following the viral success story of Sumiko Watanabe and her husband Hitoshi Watanabe, which was shared on a prominent Japanese social networking site in 2008. The diet was not devised by nutritionists or health specialists, but rather developed via the couple's personal experience and their endeavor to discover a straightforward and efficient method for weight loss.

• Sumiko Watanabe, a pharmacist, and her husband Hitoshi Watanabe, a preventive medicine expert, devised the diet plan based on their personal experience of losing weight. The primary component of the diet regimen was the ingestion of bananas during the morning meal, as they held the belief that this practice had a significant role in their achievement of weight reduction. The diet had a surge in popularity after being showcased in the media and internet forums, prompting many individuals to embrace it because of its perceived simplicity and the amazing change of the pair.

• The Morning Banana Diet gained popularity at the same time as the release of a book called "The Morning Banana Diet" (known as "Asa Banana Diet" in Japanese), authored by Sumiko Watanabe. The book delineated the couple's experiences and expounded upon the ideas of the diet, so augmenting its appeal.

• Although the Morning Banana Diet garnered a significant number of followers, it is important to emphasize that its roots are not based on scientific study or professional nutritional guidance. Like other popular diets, the Morning Banana Diet can have different effects on individuals and may not be appropriate for everyone. Prior to making any substantial dietary modifications, it is recommended to get guidance from healthcare specialists or certified dietitians.

Preparing Mentally and Physically

Prior to embarking on any diet, such as the Morning Banana Diet, it is crucial to adequately prepare oneself both emotionally and physically in order to achieve sustained success. Here are some suggestions to assist you in preparing:

Cognitively:

• **Establish Pragmatic Expectations:** Recognize that there is no universal diet that yields identical results for every individual. Establish pragmatic expectations for your objectives and acknowledge that enduring transformations require a considerable amount of time.

• **Adopt a positive mindset:** Approach the diet with an optimistic attitude. Direct your attention towards the prospective advantages for your health and enhancements, rather than merely focusing on shedding pounds.

• **Acquire knowledge:** Familiarize yourself with the ideas and criteria of the Morning Banana Diet. Gaining insight into the rationale behind specific recommendations might strengthen your dedication and comprehension.

• Practice mindful eating by fully embracing the notion. Be mindful of your body's signals for hunger and fullness, and take pleasure in each mouthful. Refrain from hastily consuming food.

• Analyze emotional factors that may contribute to the development of harmful eating patterns. Formulate alternate methods of dealing with stress and develop strategies for managing it.

• Consider maintaining a food journal or diary to record your meals, emotions, and any difficulties you have. Utilizing this tool can assist you in recognizing recurring trends and implementing well-informed modifications.

- **Establish a Support System:** Communicate your objectives to friends or family members, or contemplate seeking a diet companion. Having a network of people who provide support can serve as a source of incentive and responsibility.

- **Adaptability:** Remain receptive to modifying the diet to suit your way of life. It is permissible to make alterations that align with your personal preferences and requirements.

In Terms Of the Body:

• **Seek advice from an Expert:** Prior to embarking on any novel dietary regimen, particularly if one possesses preexisting health concerns, it is advisable to get guidance from a healthcare practitioner or a certified nutritionist. They can offer tailored guidance based on your current health condition.

• **Meal Planning:** Prearrange your meals. Implementing a meal plan facilitates the selection of healthy foods and diminishes the probability of succumbing to impulsive, less nourishing alternatives.

• **Acquire Sufficient Stock:** Make sure you have an abundant quantity of bananas and other suggested food items. Having easily accessible and appropriate ingredients facilitates adherence to the diet.

• Enhance your hydration by increasing your consumption of water. Maintaining proper hydration is essential for general well-being and can aid in managing appetite. It is advisable to carry a water bottle with you at all times.

• Integrate low-impact physical activity into your daily schedule. These activities could include walking, doing yoga, or engaging in other enjoyable physical exercises. Physical activity enhances one's overall state of health and might support one's dietary endeavors.

• Emphasize the need of maintaining good sleep hygiene. Make sure you are obtaining a enough amount of high-quality sleep every night, since it has a substantial impact on both your overall health and your ability to manage your weight.

It is important to note that the Morning Banana Diet may not be appropriate for all individuals, and it is essential to prioritize total well-being rather than only concentrating on weight reduction. Pay close attention to the signals your body is sending, make necessary modifications, and maintain a patient attitude towards the progress.

CHAPTER TWO
Getting Started Morning Banana Diet

If you have a desire to experiment with the Morning Banana Diet, here are a few instructions to assist you in commencing the regimen:

1. Comprehend the fundamental principles: Acquaint yourself with the fundamental concepts of the Morning Banana Diet, which often involve having one or more bananas for breakfast, waiting for 15 minutes before eating additional foods, and taking a more laid-back approach to meals throughout the day.

2. Strategize Your Breakfast: Ensure that you have ripe bananas readily available. You have the option to consume them in their natural state or integrate them into a basic meal, such as by slicing them onto whole-grain toast or blending them into yogurt. Ensure that you consume the bananas at the optimal ambient temperature.

3. Adhere to Guidelines for Other Meals: Although there are no rigid regulations for lunch and supper, strive for well-balanced and reasonable meals. Cease consumption when you have a sense of satisfaction, as opposed to a state of excessive fullness. The diet promotes conscientious and regulated consumption of food. It is advisable to include a diverse range of fruits, vegetables, lean proteins, and whole grains in your meals.

4. Refrain from indulging in late-night snacking by strictly following the rule of abstaining from consuming any food after 8 PM. This method is said to enable your digestive system to undergo a period of rest during the night.

5. Maintain proper hydration by consuming water regularly throughout the day. The diet suggests consuming water at a moderate temperature, either room temperature or lukewarm.

6. Take into account sleep and lifestyle factors: Strive to obtain 7-8 hours of sleep each night, as sleep is regarded as a crucial component of the Morning Banana Diet. Furthermore, endeavor to handle stress and integrate low-impact physical activity into your daily schedule if preferred.

7. Maintain A Record Of Your Progress: Contemplate maintaining a notebook to monitor your meals, your emotional state, and any alterations in your weight or overall state of health. This might aid in evaluating the efficacy of the diet for your specific requirements.

8. Maintain adaptability: Although the Morning Banana Diet offers instructions, it is crucial to remain flexible and heed the signals your body sends. If you experience lingering hunger after breakfast, it is advisable to delay your decision to eat more or go to the next meal for a period of 15 minutes.

9. Seek advice from a healthcare professional: Prior to initiating any new dietary regimen or implementing substantial modifications to your eating patterns, it is recommended to consult with a healthcare practitioner or a qualified dietitian. They are capable of offering tailored guidance according to your current health condition and specific requirements.

Please be aware that the Morning Banana Diet may not be suitable for all individuals, and personal experiences may differ. Emphasizing holistic health and well-being should take precedence over exclusively concentrating on weight reduction.

The Banana as a Super food

Although there is no precise scientific meaning for the phrase "superfood," it is commonly employed to refer to meals that are rich in nutrients and offer various health advantages. Due to their nutritional composition and the numerous beneficial impacts they can have on health, bananas are frequently regarded as a superfood. There are several reasons why bananas are commonly considered a superfood:

- **Abundant in Nutrients:** Bananas are a rich source of vital nutrients, including potassium, vitamin C, vitamin B6, and dietary fiber. These nutrients have essential functions in preserving general well-being, bolstering the immune system, and facilitating appropriate digestion.

- Bananas are renowned for their elevated potassium levels. Potassium is vital for cardiovascular well-being, muscular performance, and the maintenance of optimal fluid equilibrium inside the body. Sufficient consumption of potassium is linked to a reduced likelihood of stroke and can aid in the control of blood pressure.

• Bananas are rich in natural sugars, specifically fructose, glucose, and sucrose, which serve as a rapid and easily digestible energy source. As a result, they are frequently chosen as a pre-workout or lunchtime snack.

• Bananas promote digestive health by containing dietary fiber, especially soluble fiber, which aids in regulating bowel movements and maintaining a healthy digestive tract. Bananas are frequently suggested for those experiencing stomach problems.

• Bananas promote heart health by regulating blood pressure, mitigating the risk of cardiovascular illnesses, and boosting overall cardiovascular function due to their potassium, fiber, and antioxidants content.

• Bananas possess a variety of antioxidants, including as dopamine and catechins. Antioxidants aid in the neutralization of detrimental free radicals within the body, safeguarding cells from oxidative stress and inflammation.

• Bananas are a natural mood enhancer because they contain tryptophan, an amino acid that helps produce serotonin. Serotonin is a neurotransmitter that is linked to the control of mood and can produce a relaxing and mood-enhancing impact.

- **Weight Management:** Despite its relatively modest calorie content, bananas are satiating and can aid in suppressing cravings. The presence of dietary fiber facilitates satiety, potentially assisting in the regulation of body weight.

- Bananas has versatility and accessibility as they are convenient, portable, and do not necessitate any preparation. They are readily available throughout the year, making them a convenient and versatile addition to many dietary plans.

It is crucial to acknowledge that although bananas provide multiple health advantages, maintaining a well-rounded diet that incorporates a diverse range of fruits, vegetables, healthy grains, and proteins is essential for general wellness. Furthermore, it is recommended to seek specialized dietary guidance from a healthcare practitioner or a qualified dietitian, as individual nutritional requirements can differ.

CHAPTER THREE
Nutritional Benefits

Bananas offer a range of nutritional benefits, making them a popular and healthy fruit choice. Here are some of the key nutritional benefits of bananas:

• **Rich in Potassium:** Bananas are well-known for their high potassium content. Potassium is an essential mineral that plays a crucial role in maintaining proper heart and muscle function, regulating fluid balance, and supporting nerve signals.

• **Good Source of Vitamins:** Bananas contain various vitamins, including vitamin C, vitamin B6, and small amounts of other B vitamins. Vitamin

C is an antioxidant that supports the immune system, while vitamin B6 is essential for brain development and function.

• **Dietary Fiber:** Bananas are a good source of dietary fiber, with both soluble and insoluble fibers. Fiber supports digestive health by promoting regular bowel movements, preventing constipation, and contributing to a feeling of fullness.

• **Natural Sugars:** Bananas contain natural sugars, including fructose, glucose, and sucrose. These sugars provide a quick and easily digestible source of energy, making bananas an excellent choice for a natural energy boost.

- **Antioxidants:** Bananas contain various antioxidants, including dopamine and catechins. Antioxidants help neutralize free radicals in the body, protecting cells from oxidative stress and inflammation.

- **Low in Calories and Fat:** Bananas are relatively low in calories and fat, making them a healthy and satisfying snack option. They can be included in weight management and balanced diet plans.

- **Supportive of Heart Health:** The potassium and fiber in bananas contribute to heart health. Potassium helps regulate blood pressure, while fiber can assist in managing cholesterol levels.

- **Natural Mood Enhancer:** Bananas contain tryptophan, an amino acid that contributes to the production of serotonin. Serotonin is a neurotransmitter associated with mood regulation, potentially providing a natural mood-enhancing effect.

- **Convenient and Portable:** Bananas are easy to carry and require no preparation, making them a convenient and portable snack option. Their accessibility makes it simple to incorporate them into various diets and lifestyles.

- **Hydration:** Bananas have a high water content, contributing to hydration. Staying hydrated is crucial for overall health, and consuming water-rich fruits like bananas can be part of maintaining proper fluid balance.

It's important to note that while bananas offer these nutritional benefits, a well-rounded and diverse diet that includes a variety of fruits, vegetables, whole grains, and proteins is essential for optimal health. Individual nutritional needs may vary, so it's advisable to consult with a healthcare professional or a registered dietitian for personalized dietary advice.

Meal Planning

Meal planning is a very efficient approach for maintaining organization, optimizing time management, and selecting healthier food options. Below is a systematic strategy to assist you in meal planning:

• Establish your objectives and preferences: Assess your nutritional objectives, dietary inclinations, and any dietary limitations or food sensitivities. Take into account variables such as weight control, medical issues, financial resources, and culinary abilities.

• Establish a weekly schedule for meals: Utilize a calendar or meal planning application to delineate your meals for the entire week. Please provide meals for breakfast, lunch, dinner, and snacks. It is advisable to include the practice of preparing extra food or cooking in large quantities in order to save time.

• Select recipes that correspond to your objectives and personal tastes. Seek out well-balanced meals that incorporate a diverse range of essential nutrients, such as lean proteins, whole grains, beneficial fats, and ample amounts of fruits and vegetables. Incorporate a selection of your preferred foods to enhance the pleasure of eating.

• **Generate a Shopping List:** Utilizing the recipes you have selected, compile a comprehensive list of the necessary ingredients required for the upcoming week. Categorize the list according to food groups (such as produce, dairy, and pantry essentials) in order to enhance shopping efficiency. Inspect your kitchen for existing products to prevent unnecessary expenditures.

• Prepare materials: Allocate a portion of time to preparing materials beforehand, such as cleansing and dicing vegetables, marinating meats, or boiling grains and legumes. Preparing ingredients in advance facilitates the process of assembling meals, saving time and effort, especially on hectic weekdays.

• Employ batch cooking or prepare greater quantities of specific dishes that can be divided into portions and consumed over the course of the week. Batch cooking is best suited for preparing soups, stews, casseroles, and grain-based salads.

• **Embrace adaptability:** Incorporate flexibility into your meal plan to suit alterations in your schedule, unforeseen circumstances, or impromptu desires. Ensure that you have a repertoire of convenient and effortless meal suggestions available for those busy days when preparing meals from scratch is not practical.

- **Utilize leftover food efficiently:** Intend to transform leftover food into fresh meals in order to reduce food waste. As an illustration, you can roast additional vegetables to include them into salads or omelets, or repurpose any remaining grilled chicken by making tacos or wraps.

- **Maintain organization:** Store your meal plan, recipes, and shopping list in a centralized spot, such as a meal planning notebook or a digital application. Consistently assess and revise your meal plan to accurately reflect alterations in personal tastes or the seasonal accessibility of ingredients.

- **Embrace diversity:** Strive for diversity in your meals to guarantee a broad spectrum of nutrients and flavors. Engage in culinary experimentation by exploring novel dishes, diverse cuisines, and unfamiliar ingredients to maintain a sense of excitement and pleasure in your meals.

Keep in mind that meal planning is a flexible procedure, so discover a technique that suits you and your way of life most effectively. Through regular practice and unwavering commitment, meal planning can evolve into a vital instrument for upholding a nourishing and well-rounded diet.

CHAPTER FOUR
Exercise and Physical Activity

Exercise and physical exercise are essential elements of a healthy lifestyle, providing a multitude of advantages for both physical and mental health. Here are crucial factors to contemplate while integrating exercise into your daily regimen:

Categories of Physical Activity:

1. Cardiovascular Exercise:

• **Definition:** Physical activities that increase your heart rate and enhance cardiovascular well-being.

• Examples of physical activities include running, brisk walking, cycling, swimming, and dancing.

2. Strength Training:

- **Definition:** Physical exercises that utilize resistance in order to enhance muscle strength and endurance.

- Examples of exercises include weightlifting, bodyweight exercises such as push-ups and squats, and resistance band workouts.

3. Flexibility and Stretching:

- **Definition:** Exercises that enhance flexibility and the ability to move joints through their full range of motion.

- Examples of activities that fall under this category include yoga, Pilates, and static stretching.

4. Balance and Stability Training:

• **Definition:** Exercises designed to improve balance and stability.

• Examples of exercises that improve balance include balance exercises and stability ball workouts.

The Advantages Of Physical Activity:

1. Physical Health:

• **Cardiovascular Health:** Decreases the likelihood of developing heart disease, reduces blood pressure, and enhances blood flow.

• **Weight Management:** Facilitates weight loss or maintenance through calorie expenditure.

Strength training enhances muscle and bone density, promoting muscle and bone health.

2. Mental Health:

• **Tension Reduction:** The act of releasing endorphins helps to alleviate tension and anxiety.

• **Enhanced Mood:** Elevates mood and counteracts signs of depression.

Regular exercise might enhance the quality of sleep.

3. Overall Well-Being:

• **Enhanced Vitality:** Elevates energy levels and alleviates tiredness.

Regular exercise has the ability to fortify the immune system, resulting in an enhanced level of immunity.

• **Enhanced Cognitive Function:** Enhances brain health and cognitive function.

Guidelines for Commencing:

1. Establish Attainable Objectives:

• Begin with realistic goals and incrementally advance as your physical fitness enhances.

2. Opt for activities that you derive pleasure from in order to enhance the probability of maintaining consistency with them.

3. Commence at A Leisurely Pace:

• If you are inexperienced in physical activity, initiate with low-intensity exercises and progressively escalate the level of exertion and length of time.

4. Diversify your workout regimen by include a range of workouts that target various muscle groups, ensuring both effectiveness and engagement.

5. Place emphasis on Consistency:

• Consistency is crucial for attaining the long-term advantages of exercise. Discover a regimen that aligns with your timetable.

6. Be attuned to the signs your body sends and refrain from exerting excessive effort, particularly if you are a beginner.

7. Integrate strength training:

• Ensure to include strength training workouts at least twice a week to enhance muscle growth and boost metabolism.

8. Maintain proper hydration:

• Consume water prior to, during, and following physical activity to ensure adequate hydration.

9. Prior to engaging in physical activity, it is essential to warm up in order to prime your muscles. Similarly, after exercising, it is important to cool down in order to facilitate the recovery process.

10. Seek Expert Advice: If you have any health issues or are uncertain about the appropriate workout regimen for your needs, it is advisable to speak with a healthcare practitioner or a certified fitness trainer.

It is important to keep in mind that discovering pleasurable activities and gradually establishing a pattern that fits your lifestyle are crucial for making exercise a lasting and fulfilling aspect of your everyday life.

Overcoming Challenges

Overcoming challenges is an essential aspect of maintaining a healthy lifestyle, including sticking to an exercise routine and achieving fitness goals. Here are some strategies for overcoming common obstacles:

Lack of Motivation:

• **Set Clear Goals:** Define specific, achievable goals that inspire and motivate you.

• **Find Your Why:** Identify your reasons for wanting to exercise, whether it's improving health, reducing stress, or achieving a personal milestone.

• **Create a Routine:** Establish a consistent exercise schedule and treat it like an important appointment.

• **Mix It Up:** Keep your workouts varied and engaging by trying different activities or classes.

• **Find Accountability:** Exercise with a friend, join a group fitness class, or work with a personal trainer to stay accountable.

Time Constraints:

• **Prioritize Exercise:** Schedule workouts into your calendar just like any other important commitment.

• **Shorten Workouts:** Incorporate high-intensity interval training (HIIT) or shorter, more intense workouts when time is limited.

• **Break It Up:** Fit in shorter bursts of activity throughout the day, such as taking brisk walks during breaks or doing quick bodyweight exercises.

- **Combine Activities:** Find ways to incorporate exercise into daily tasks, such as walking or biking instead of driving, or doing household chores more vigorously.

Lack of Energy:

- **Assess Sleep Habits:** Ensure you're getting enough quality sleep each night to support energy levels.

- **Fuel Your Body:** Eat a balanced diet with nutritious foods to provide energy for workouts.

- **Pre-Workout Fuel:** Have a light snack containing carbohydrates and protein before exercising to fuel your workout.

- **Hydrate:** Drink water throughout the day to stay hydrated, as dehydration can lead to fatigue.

- **Listen to Your Body:** If you're feeling excessively tired, consider opting for a lighter workout or taking a rest day.

Plateaus and Setbacks:

- **Reevaluate Goals:** Assess your goals and adjust them if necessary to keep challenging yourself.

- **Change Your Routine:** Modify your exercise routine by increasing intensity, trying new activities, or focusing on different muscle groups.

- **Track Progress:** Keep track of your workouts, progress, and achievements to stay motivated and recognize improvements.

- **Practice Patience:** Plateaus are a normal part of the fitness journey. Stay consistent and trust the process, knowing that progress takes time.

Lack of Resources or Access:

- **Explore Affordable Options:** Look for free or low-cost fitness resources, such as community centers, outdoor spaces, or online workout videos.

- **Get Creative:** Use household items as makeshift weights, or take advantage of bodyweight exercises that require minimal equipment.

- **Utilize Technology:** Explore fitness apps, YouTube channels, or virtual classes for guided workouts that can be done from home.

• **Seek Community Support:** Connect with others who share similar fitness goals through online forums, social media groups, or local fitness communities.

Injury or Health Concerns:

• **Listen to Your Body:** Pay attention to any signs of discomfort or pain during exercise, and adjust your routine accordingly.

• **Consult a Professional:** Seek guidance from a healthcare professional or physical therapist if you're dealing with an injury or health condition. They can provide personalized advice and rehabilitation exercises.

• **Focus on Recovery:** Allow your body adequate time to rest and recover from workouts, and incorporate activities like stretching, foam rolling, or yoga to improve flexibility and prevent injury.

By implementing these strategies and staying committed to your fitness journey, you can overcome common challenges and continue progressing toward your goals. Remember that consistency, perseverance, and flexibility are key to long-term success.

Maintaining the Morning Banana Diet

Maintaining the Morning Banana Diet or any dietary regimen requires commitment, consistency, and adaptability. Here's how you can effectively maintain the Morning Banana Diet:

Establish a Routine:

• **Consistent Breakfast:** Make eating bananas for breakfast a daily habit. Choose ripe bananas and consume them at room temperature as recommended.

• **Meal Structure:** Follow the guidelines of the Morning Banana Diet, such as waiting 15 minutes before consuming other foods after eating bananas for breakfast and avoiding late-night snacking.

• **Mindful Eating:** Practice mindful eating throughout the day, focusing on listening to your body's hunger and fullness cues. Eat slowly and savor each bite to promote satisfaction and prevent overeating.

Plan and Prepare:

• **Meal Planning:** Plan your meals and snacks around the Morning Banana Diet's principles. Incorporate a variety of nutrient-dense foods to ensure balanced nutrition.

• **Stock Up on Bananas:** Keep a supply of ripe bananas on hand so you're always prepared for breakfast. Consider buying in bulk and freezing extra bananas for smoothies or baking.

• **Prep Healthy Snacks:** Have healthy snack options readily available, such as cut-up fruits, vegetables, nuts, or yogurt, to prevent reaching for unhealthy choices when hunger strikes.

Stay Hydrated:

• **Water Intake:** Drink plenty of water throughout the day, as staying hydrated is essential for overall health and can help control appetite.

• **Herbal Teas:** Enjoy herbal teas as an alternative to sugary or caffeinated beverages. Herbal teas can provide hydration and contribute to feelings of relaxation and well-being.

Incorporate Physical Activity:

• **Regular Exercise:** Include regular physical activity in your routine to complement the Morning Banana Diet. Aim for a combination of cardiovascular exercise, strength training, flexibility, and balance exercises.

• **Find Enjoyable Activities:** Choose physical activities that you enjoy and look forward to, whether it's walking, cycling, dancing, or participating in group fitness classes.

Listen to Your Body:

- **Self-awareness:** Pay attention to how your body responds to the Morning Banana Diet. Adjust your eating habits, portion sizes, and meal timing based on your hunger levels, energy levels, and overall well-being.

- **Flexibility:** Be flexible and adaptable with your dietary choices. While bananas are the cornerstone of the diet, allow yourself the freedom to enjoy a variety of foods that nourish your body and satisfy your taste preferences.

Seek Support and Accountability:

- **Community:** Connect with others who follow the Morning Banana Diet or have similar health goals. Share experiences, recipes, and tips for staying motivated and on track.

- **Accountability Partner:** Partner with a friend, family member, or online accountability group to support each other in maintaining healthy eating habits and staying committed to your goals.

Monitor Progress and Celebrate Success:

- **Track Your Journey:** Keep a journal to record your meals, exercise, mood, and progress. Reflect on your achievements, challenges, and areas for improvement.

- **Celebrate Milestones:** Acknowledge and celebrate your achievements, whether it's reaching a weight loss goal, improving fitness levels, or developing healthier eating habits.

By incorporating these strategies into your lifestyle, you can effectively maintain the Morning Banana Diet and promote long-term health and well-being. Remember to approach dietary changes with patience, consistency, and a focus on overall balance and sustainability.

Conclusion

In conclusion, the Morning Banana Diet gained popularity as a simple and flexible approach to weight management and overall well-being. While its origins are rooted in the personal experiences of a Japanese couple, Sumiko and Hitoshi Watanabe, its widespread adoption highlights the appeal of a straightforward and accessible dietary plan.

The key principles of the Morning Banana Diet involve starting the day with one or more bananas for breakfast, waiting 15 minutes before consuming other foods, and adopting a mindful and balanced approach to meals throughout the day. The diet emphasizes the importance of hydration, regular sleep, and gentle exercise.

While bananas are recognized as a nutrient-dense fruit with various health benefits, it's crucial to approach the Morning Banana Diet with a realistic understanding of its potential impact. Individual responses to dietary plans can vary, and it's advisable to consult with healthcare professionals or registered dietitians before making significant changes to one's eating habits.

Ultimately, maintaining the Morning Banana Diet or any dietary regimen requires a combination of commitment, consistency, and adaptability. It's important to listen to your body, make adjustments as needed, and prioritize overall health and well-being. A holistic approach that includes a variety of nutrient-rich foods, regular physical activity, and mindful eating practices can contribute to sustainable and positive lifestyle changes.

THE END